HEALTH SCIENCE

Active Health Investigations

Science Action Labs

Written by Edward Shevick
Illustrated by Marguerite Jones

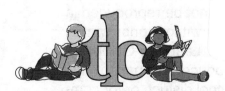

Teaching & Learning Company

1204 Buchanan St., P.O. Box 10
Carthage, IL 62321-0010

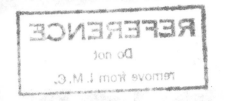

This book belongs to

_____

Cover by Marguerite Jones

Copyright © 1998, Teaching & Learning Company

ISBN No. 1-57310-143-5

Printing No. 987654321

Teaching & Learning Company
1204 Buchanan St., P.O. Box 10
Carthage, IL 62321-0010

TLC10143 Copyright © Teaching & Learning Company, Carthage, IL 62321-0010

Table of Contents
Science Action Labs

Dear Teacher or Parent,

This book is about the human body. It is for students and teachers who want to be actively involved in health education. Only a small portion of this book explains the science of the body. Most of the book involves fun activities that will teach your students how their bodies work.

Health Science uses the spirit of Sir Isaac Newton to provide background and motivation. This health book uses an imaginary descendant of Sir Isaac Newton to guide you. His name is Dr. G.H. Newton. G and H stand for *good health*.

This book can help your students in many ways. Choose some activities to spice up your class. Most sections can be converted to hands-on lab activities for the entire class. Some can be developed into student projects or reports. Every class has a few students with a special zest for health science. Encourage them to pursue some health science activities on their own.

The answers you will need are on page 64.

Your students will get more out of this book if you follow these health science guidelines:

1. **Observe carefully.**
2. **Follow directions.**
3. **Measure carefully.**
4. **Hypothesize intelligently.**
5. **Experiment safely.**
6. **Keep experimenting until you succeed.**

Sincerely,

Ed

Edward Shevick

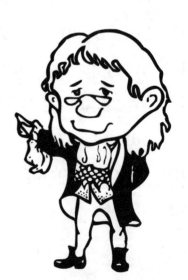

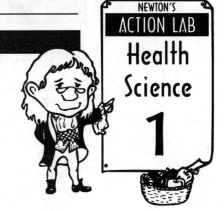

Health Superstitions

Dr. Newton Wants You to Know

Throughout the ages, people have held false beliefs about many things including diseases, animals and the sun. These false, unfounded beliefs are called **superstitions**. Superstitions are not based upon careful observations, measurements, experiments or logical thinking. They are usually based upon fear, ignorance, prejudice and careless observations.

People once had many false ideas about blood. They believed that blood left the heart, oozed through the body and passed through the pores of the skin. William Harvey used science to prove that blood circulates around the body. In fact, blood can race from your heart to your toes and back to your heart in one minute.

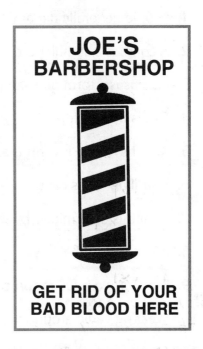

JOE'S
BARBERSHOP

GET RID OF YOUR
BAD BLOOD HERE

Not long ago a sick person was considered to have "bad" blood. The cure was to cut the patient to allow the poisoned blood to leave the body. This blood letting was done by barbers. The red stripes on modern barbershop poles are reminders of this old false belief. It took science, not superstition, to discover the importance of blood in fighting disease.

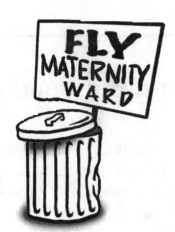

FLY
MATERNITY
WARD

Once upon a time people believed that garbage gave "birth" to flies. They observed that worms, called maggots, appeared on garbage and developed into flies. It seemed logical that somehow the garbage was responsible for flies. It wasn't until 1668 that Francesco Redi applied the scientific method to the problem. His experiments proved that the maggots really came from eggs laid by adult flies.

Name _____

Sharing Superstitions

You'll find a short list of health superstitions below. Check with your friends to find how many people believe in them.

Ask your parents or grandparents to tell you about any health superstitions that they may have had when they were growing up.

1. People generally die at the same age as their parents.

2. Alcohol is a stimulant to your body.

3. Genius is a form of insanity.

4. Fish is a brain food.

5. Men have one less rib than women.

6. Handling toads causes warts on your skin.

7. Health is determined by the stars under which you are born.

8. Night air is unhealthy.

9. Exposure to a full moon can affect your mental health.

10. Wearing garlic around your neck keeps you healthy.

11. Eating food cooked in aluminum can harm you.

12. Birthmarks are caused by a shock to the mother before birth.

13. Flowers and plants should be removed from a hospital room at night.

14. The author has added a fourteenth superstition because the number 13 is supposed to be unlucky.

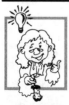

Dr. Newton Wants You to Avoid Quacks

A **quack** is someone who falsely promotes medical products or services. You wouldn't buy skunk oil to cure cancer or baldness. Yet, down through the ages, people have been taken in by quacks and their phony cures. Even today, it is estimated that Americans pay over a billion dollars yearly to medical quacks.

Name _____

Dr. Newton wants you to learn more about quacks by joining them! Combine with others to develop a complete sales campaign for a **phony health product**. Do such a great job that you might want to use the product yourself.

1. Decide on one quack device or product to promote. The partial list below can be used or you can choose your own.

2. Construct a "gimmick." This can be a huge model pill, a fake electronic device, a food package or "?".

3. Design a full-page ad to be placed in a national magazine. Before you decide on the layout of your ad, study magazine ads to determine how to have maximum emotional appeal.

4. Feel free to use partial truths, references to false authorities, testimonials from cured people, hints about mysterious qualities or powers and money-back guarantees.

5. Prepare a two-minute TV commercial. Observe real TV commercials carefully to see how they get maximum "sell" into a short period of time.

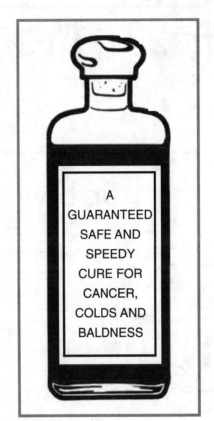

A GUARANTEED SAFE AND SPEEDY CURE FOR CANCER, COLDS AND BALDNESS

Quack product suggestions (use these or your own quack ideas):

liver pills	smoking cures
blood purifiers	electronic healing machines
skin foods	youth restorers
weight loss products	I.Q. raising pills
cancer-curing chemicals	hair-growing creams

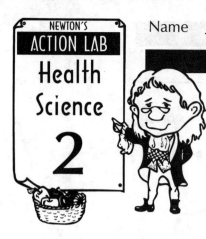

Name _____

Man's Marvelous Machine

Dr. Newton Wants You to Know

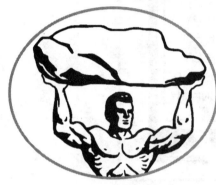

Your most precious possession is your body. Compare your body to a rock. You grow, but a rock doesn't. You breathe, but a rock doesn't. You think, but a rock doesn't.

Each sentence below tells something about **living** things such as your body. The key word in each sentence has been scrambled. Unscramble the bold-faced word and write it correctly. Study the example for help.

LIVING SENTENCES	UNSCRAMBLED WORD
Example: Living things **PROREEDUC**.	Example: **REPRODUCE**
1. Living things need **RAI**.	1. _ _ _
2. Living things **OVEM**.	2. _ _ _ _
3. Living things **WGRO**.	3. _ _ _ _
4. Living things need **ODOF**.	4. _ _ _ _
5. Living things **IDE**.	5. _ _ _
6. Living things have definite **ZIES**.	6. _ _ _ _
7. Living things **TACER** to the world around them.	7. _ _ _ _ _
8. Living things need **TWARE**.	8. _ _ _ _ _
9. Living things give off **STEWA** materials.	9. _ _ _ _ _
10. Living things can **PRAIRE** themselves.	10. _ _ _ _ _ _
11. Living things are made of **SLECL**.	11. _ _ _ _ _
12. **TOPSLAMORP** is the basic ingredient in all living cells.	12. _ _ _ _ _ _ _ _ _ _

8

TLC10143 Copyright © Teaching & Learning Company, Carthage, IL 62321-0010

Name _____

How Long Can It Live?

Every living thing has a normal life expectancy. Sequoia redwood trees can live over 4000 years. Human life expectancy has increased dramatically in recent years. Yet, it is still much higher in some countries than others.

Dr. Newton wants you to take this guessing game. It compares the life expectancy of humans and other animals. Make your **best guess** in the column provided.

LIFE EXPECTANCY – HOW LONG DO YOU THINK THEY LIVE?				
	Your Guess			Your Guess
1. fly		10. man born in 1770 (George Washington's time)		
2. mouse		11. man born in 1900		
3. dog		12. child born at this moment in India		
4. cat		13. child born at this moment in Mexico		
5. horse		14. child born at this moment in Sweden		
6. elephant		15. male child born at this moment in USA		
7. tortoise		16. female child born at this moment in USA		
8. eagle		17. male child born at this moment in Kenya, Africa		
9. goldfish				

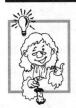

Dr. Newton Wants You to Go Further

Check with all your friends. Who has the oldest grandfather? Who has the oldest grandmother?

Contact a local senior citizens' home. You will be surprised at how happy they are to speak to young people. Have them give you the total number of seniors in the home and the breakdown into how many men and women. The greater number of women will amaze you. Can you think of three good reasons why women live longer?

UNITED STATES POPULATION FACTS

- There are 262,000,000 plus people in the United States.
- A child is born every eight seconds.
- Someone dies every 13 seconds.
- Someone immigrates into the United States every 37 seconds.
- Someone moves from the United States every 198 seconds.

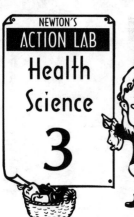

Name _____

Your Growing Body

Dr. Newton Wants You to Know

Look carefully at your friends. You and your friends are all classified by scientists as *Homo sapiens*. This means you are similar to other mammals, similar to other primates (monkeys) and are man-like (Homo) with sense (*sapiens*). You and your friends are much more alike than you are different. You are still very different in height, weight and body proportions.

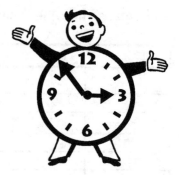

WORLD RECORDS FOR HUMAN SIZE

Tallest man:
Robert Wadlow; 8 feet, 11.1 inches

Tallest woman:
Jane Bunford; 7 feet, 11 inches

Smallest person:
Pauline Musters, 23.2 inches and
9 pounds at age 19

Heaviest man:
Robert Hughes, 1069 pounds

Heaviest woman:
Pearl Washington, 880 pounds

Differences are determined by your heredity, your environment and by a "biological clock" inside of you that controls the timing and rate of your growth. You can understand how important this "biological clock" is by considering that a baby weighs about 7 pounds (3 kg) at birth and triples its weight to about 21 pounds (9 kg) in one year. Imagine what you would look like at ages 2, 3 and up if the biological clock did not slow up your growth rate.

Your Changing Body

You Are Not as Tall at Night

You have changed a lot since you were a baby. You will change more as you eventually become a senior citizen. Strangely enough, you even change height every day.

1. Measure your height accurately first thing in the morning. _____ inches (cm)

2. Measure your height accurately again just before bedtime. _____ inches (cm)

3. How much did you shrink by bedtime? _____ inches (cm)

10

Your Growing Body

Name _____

Your backbone has many bones separated by soft cartilage discs that act as cushions. Standing all day squeezes the cushioning discs together.

Head to Body Proportions

It is obvious that a baby's head is quite large compared to its body length. The average baby's head is usually about one-fourth of the total baby length.

In this activity you are encouraged to collect head and body data from as many people as possible. Try infants, boys, girls, men, women and senior citizens. There is a data table below to guide you.

1. Collect age, head size and total height from as many people as possible.

2. Use **caution** and get parents' permission when measuring small children.

3. Measure total height in inches. **Round off to the nearest inch**.

4. Measure head length from the tip of the chin to the top of the scalp. Don't count hair.

5. Use a calculator to divide head height by total height. This will help you get the percent. **Round off all measurements to the nearest inch or percent**. You don't have to be super accurate.

SUBJECT NAME	AGE	A HEAD LENGTH INCHES	B TOTAL HEIGHT INCHES	$\frac{A}{B}$ = $\frac{HEAD}{HEIGHT}$ = %
1. Example: Bill Jones	40	9	69	$\frac{9}{69}$ = .13 = 13%
2.				
3.				
4.				
5.				
6.				
7.				

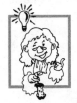

Predicting Your Adult Height and Weight

The *average* American male is about 5' 10" (178 cm) tall and weighs 155 pounds (70 kg). The *average* American female is about 5' 4" (163 cm) tall and weighs about 128 pounds (58 kg).

How much will you weigh and how tall will you be when you mature? Nobody knows for sure. However, you can use the formulas on page 12 to make a **rough** prediction.

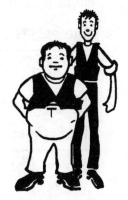

Your Growing Body

Name ______________________________

1. Measure your height to the **nearest** inch. __________ inches
2. Measure your weight to the **nearest** pound. __________ pounds
3. Pick your age out of the **boy** or **girl** data table and prepare to do some simple math.

BOY TABLE

Between Ages	% OF FINAL HEIGHT	% OF FINAL WEIGHT
11-12	80%	56%
12-13	87%	62%
13-14	90%	69%
14-15	95%	87%

GIRL TABLE

Between Ages	% OF FINAL HEIGHT	% OF FINAL WEIGHT
11-12	88%	68%
12-13	92%	78%
13-14	95%	87%
14-15	98%	95%

Sample Problem: Assume a boy between 13 and 14 years of age is 65 inches tall and weighs 120 pounds.

1. His predicted future height =

$$\frac{\text{present height in inches x 100}}{\text{\% from table}} \quad X \quad \frac{65 \times 100}{90\%} = \frac{6500}{90} = \text{72 inches}$$

2. His predicted future weight =

$$\frac{\text{present weight in pounds x 100}}{\text{\% from table}} \quad X \quad \frac{120 \times 100}{69\%} = \frac{12{,}000}{69} = \text{174 pounds}$$

Name _____

1. Try to predict your future height and weight.

2. Try to predict the future height and weight of some of your friends. Don't take the prediction results too seriously. There is no perfect formula.

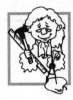

Dr. Newton Wants to Check Your Weight

Humans come in all sizes and shapes. Yet, there is a normal size and shape for most people depending on both their heredity and environment.

Dr. Newton has worked out a method of finding how "normal" your present weight is without using a scale. All you have to do is use a string or tape measure to find your **height** and **waist** size.

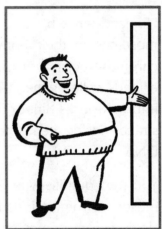

1. Measure your height in inches. Round off to the nearest inch. _____ inches

2. Measure your waist in inches at the thickest part. _____ inches

3. Simple math. Subtract the waist measurement from your height measurement. _____ Answer

Use Dr. Newton's scale below to see if you are too slim or too chubby. Don't take the results too seriously.

Example: A 70-inch tall person with a 37-inch waist.

70 - 37 = 33

Use Dr. Newton's scale below to see if you are too slim or too chubby. Again, don't take the results too seriously.

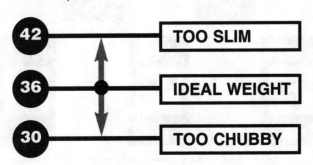

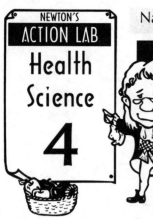

Heredity: Thank Your Parents

Dr. Newton Wants You to Know

Human beings have 23 pairs of **chromosomes** in their body cells. Each chromosome, in turn, is made of smaller parts called **genes**. The hereditary information is lined up in twisted strands inside genes that are called DNA.

You start out life with 23 single chromosomes from your dad and 23 more single chromosomes from your mom. These combine to make you a normal human being with 23 **pairs** of genes. These genes can combine in many ways to make you different from all other human beings. Scientists claim that a set of parents would need to give birth to 70 trillion children before having two that are exactly alike.

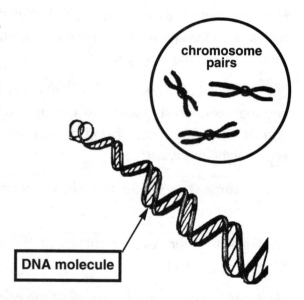

chromosome pairs

DNA molecule

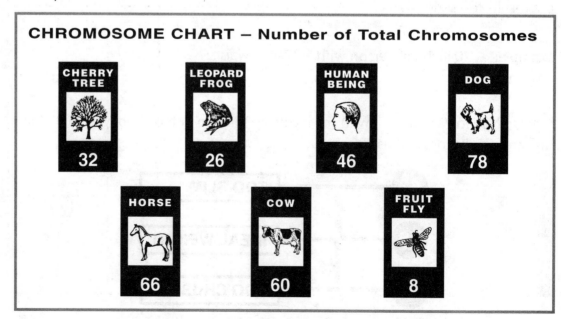

CHROMOSOME CHART – Number of Total Chromosomes

CHERRY TREE	LEOPARD FROG	HUMAN BEING	DOG
32	26	46	78

HORSE	COW	FRUIT FLY
66	60	8

Name _____

Your Family Tree

Take a good look at your family. You will probably see many more resemblances than differences. You are part of a vast pool of inherited genes that go back way beyond your grandparents. Be prepared to find great variety in your family features.

You are now about to fill out a chart of family traits that you may or may not have inherited. Be mature. Don't take the results too seriously. Predicting inherited traits is difficult even for scientists.

FAMILY TRAIT CHART

	TRAIT	INSTRUCTIONS	ADJUST TO YOUR "OWN" FAMILY					
			You	Dad	Mom	Brother	Sister	Etc.
1	**Eye Color**	Try to give exact shade.						
2	**Hair Color**	Try to give exact shade.						
3	**Hair Curl**	Either straight or curly.						
4	**Complexion**	Light, medium or dark.						
5	**Earlobe**	Attached or free.						
6	**Finger Fold**	Put your hands together with your fingers entwined. You can have right or left thumb on top.						
7	**Finger Togetherness**	Place your left and right index fingers together with the joints even and touching firmly. The ends of your two fingers will either line up straight or form a *V*.						
8	**Tongue Curling**	Stick your tongue out and try to curl the sides up to form a *U* as shown. Seven in 10 people can curl their tongue upward, only one in 1000 can curl it downward.						
9	**Widow's Peak** PRESENT ABSENT	Record as *present* or *absent* in your family members.						

Name _____

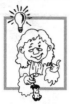

Heredity Facts and Falsehoods

There are a lot of false ideas about heredity. Some people even believe that an expectant mother should listen to good music to insure that the child will be a musician.

Here is a list of some true and some false statements about heredity. Answer true or false on each, and then check with the correct answers on page 64.

1. Identical twins are always of the same sex. _____

2. Fraternal twins look more like each other than their other brothers and sisters.

3. The father's chromosomes determine the sex of the child. _____

4. Each parent contributes half of a child's heredity. _____

5. Color blindness (which is inherited) is more common in men than women. _____

6. Inherited traits can be changed by the position at birth of stars and planets. _____

7. The tendency to produce twins runs in families. _____

8. More male than female babies are born each year. _____

9. Two brown-eyed parents can have a blue-eyed child. _____

Dr. Newton Has Some Hairy Heredity Ideas

Your hair color and whorl direction are both inherited. Check your friends and family for these traits.

Look down at someone's head. Notice that the hair forms a whorl. Some whorls are clockwise. Some are counterclockwise.

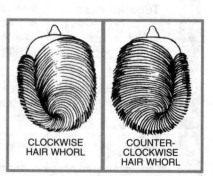

CLOCKWISE HAIR WHORL

COUNTER-CLOCKWISE HAIR WHORL

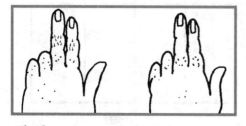

Look closely at the **middle** joints on the back of your fingers. Some people have hair on them. Some do not. Check your family and friends.

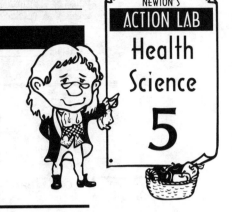

Circulating Your Blood

Dr. Newton Wants You to Know

Your blood circulates in a closed loop around your body. Every minute five quarts (4.8 l) of blood moves completely through your body. This is to insure that all your living cells are constantly bathed in blood.

WHAT BLOOD DOES

- Delivers food to the cells
- Delivers oxygen to the cells
- Removes waste materials, such as carbon dioxide, from the cells
- Circulates heat to maintain body temperature
- Fights infection
- Distributes chemicals that regulate the body

Your heart is a powerful muscular bag about the size of your fist. It is near the center of your chest cavity tilted toward the left. Your heart started beating six months before you were born. It may beat two billion times during a normal lifetime. No man-made machine can equal the heart's strength and durability. There are four sections to your heart. The upper two are called **atriums**. Blood flows *into* the atriums from the body or the lungs. The lower two sections are called **ventricles**. Ventricles pump blood out of the heart into the body or the lungs.

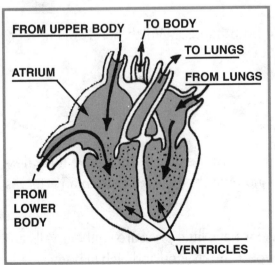

FROM UPPER BODY TO BODY TO LUNGS FROM LUNGS ATRIUM FROM LOWER BODY VENTRICLES

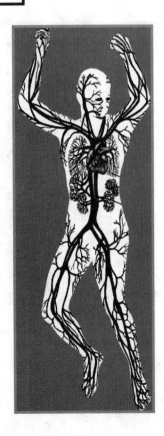

Every beat of your heart sends a spurt of blood to your body. The blood is pumped by your heart through over 60,000 miles (96,600 km) of blood vessels.

Name _____

Investigating Your Blood System

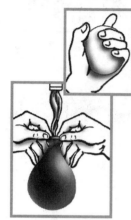

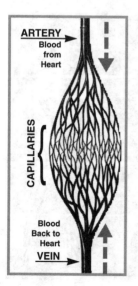

Your Heart

Your heart is basically a hollow muscle. In just one minute it can move a drop of blood from your nose to your toes and back again. Unlike other body muscles, your heart rarely rests.

1. Obtain a tennis ball.

2. Squeeze it 60 times as rapidly and vigorously as you can. This is equal to the job your heart muscle does every minute. You are fortunate that your heart muscles are stronger than your tired hand muscles.

3. Obtain a balloon and carefully fill it with water.

4. Take the water balloon **outside** or over a sink.

5. Squeeze the balloon vigorously and let the water spurt out. Your heart muscle spurts blood in the same way. Each heart contraction spurts out three ounces (89 ml) of blood at a speed of three feet (.90 m) per second.

6. Hold one hand over your head and let the other hand hang at your side for one minute.

7. After one minute, look at the back of both hands. Which hand was redder? Can you explain why?

Your Blood Tubes

Your blood system has three kinds of tubes.

1. **Arteries** are vessels that carry blood away from the heart. They have thick flexible walls to cope with the pressure found near the heart. Blood in an artery is usually rich in food and oxygen.

2. **Veins** carry blood back to the heart. Veins have little pressure so their walls are relatively thin. Blood in a vein is low in food and oxygen and high in body waste. Blood from a cut vein is dark red and flows out slowly. Veins are usually closer to the skin surface than arteries. The larger veins have cup-like valves. These valves prevent the blood from flowing backwards. Arteries do not have valves.

18

Name _____

3. **Capillaries** are tiny blood vessels that connect arteries to veins. Millions of capillaries form an intricate network. Capillary walls are only one cell thick. Materials needed by body cells can pass through these thin walls.

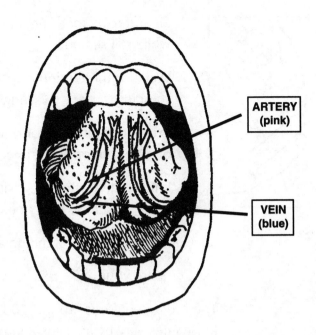

ARTERY
(pink)

VEIN
(blue)

Your tongue is a strange but useful place to observe blood tubes.

1. Use a mirror and a strong light to observe the **bottom** of your tongue. The sketch to the right will help. The two thick pink lines are arteries. The two thick blue lines are veins. You may not be able to see the much smaller capillaries. You might try observing capillaries in the fold under your eye. **Be careful**.

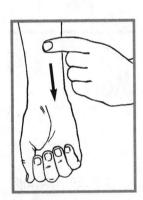

You've learned that blood flows in veins from the body back to the heart. Veins in your lower arms are close to the surface.

1. Locate a prominent vein on your or a friend's lower arm.

2. Press a finger down on the vein and keep pressing as you stroke a few inches (centimeters) toward the wrist.

3. Observe the blood flow back into the vein toward the heart as you release the pressure.

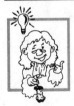

The Pulse of Life

Every beat of the heart sends a spurt of blood to your body. The rate at which your heart beats in one minute is called your **pulse**. A child's pulse is faster than an adult's. A woman's pulse is faster than a man's. Animal pulse rates can vary from 25 to 1000 per minute.

You can feel the pulse anywhere that an artery is near the surface and above a bone. You can find your pulse on your neck and your temples. Doctors usually take your pulse on the wrist.

1. Try to feel your own pulse. Press two fingers (not the thumb) on your wrist firmly. Once you feel the pulse, relax your fingers.

2. In the following pulse activities, take your own pulse or take a friend's pulse.

Name _____

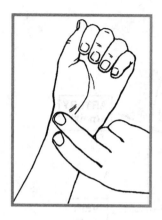

1. Sit and *relax for* three minutes. Now count your pulse beats for one minute while still seated. _____ rest beats per minute

2. Walk for three minutes. Now count your pulse beats for one minute while standing. _____ walking beats per minute

3. Exercise **vigorously** for one minute. This could be jogging in place, hopping on one foot or doing knee bends.

4. Immediately after exercising, count your pulse again for one minute. _____ exercise beats per minute

5. Compare your rest, standing and exercise pulse rates. Did they differ greatly?

6. Compare your pulse results with a friend. Did they differ?

The average pulse is around 70 beats per minute. Don't worry about your pulse. Pulse rates vary by age, sex and physical condition.

Dr. Newton Wants You to Do More

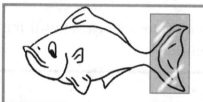

A Goldfish Tail

You can see blood flowing in a goldfish's tail. You will need a microscope, flat glass, cotton and the smallest goldfish you can buy.

1. Wrap your goldfish in wet cotton. Cover the gills, but leave the tail sticking out.

2. Place your fish on the glass. Place a smaller glass on the tail to hold it down.

3. Observe the blood flowing at the thinnest part of the tail.

4. Keep the cotton moist. Return the goldfish to its bowl every two minutes so as not to harm it.

Poetry for Your Heart

Can you use what you learned about your heart and blood to write an interesting and humorous poem? Here is a sample poem to get you started.

Around and around it goes
From the tip of my nose
To the tip of my toes
When it stops, nobody flows.

TLC10143 Copyright © Teaching & Learning Company, Carthage, IL 62321-0010

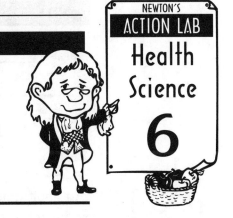

Breathing Air

Dr. Newton Wants You to Know

You can breathe through your mouth or nose. It is best to breathe through your nose. The nose has hairs that filter out dust in the air. Your nose warms and moistens the air before it gets to the lungs.

Air passes through the windpipe (trachea) on the way to the lungs. The windpipe divides into branches that serve the two lungs. Your vocal cords are at the top of the windpipe. Air must pass through the vocal cords to make sound.

1. Close your mouth, and squeeze your nose. Try to make any sound including humming. What were the results?

Your lungs are the size of footballs. They are hollow inside and have a surface area 30 times greater than your skin. Lungs exchange the oxygen your body needs with the carbon dioxide waste your body must get rid of. Blood comes to the lungs to exchange carbon dioxide for oxygen.

Twelve pairs of ribs surround and protect the soft, spongy lungs. This rib cage can expand or contract as you breathe.

2. Hold your rib cage and breathe deeply. You can feel your rib cage expand.

Lungs cannot expand and contract by themselves to move air in and out. The powerful diaphragm muscle just below the lungs causes them to move. Pulling the diaphragm muscle down fills your lungs with air. Moving the diaphragm up forces air out of your lungs.

3. Breathe in and out deeply. You can feel the diaphragm muscle move.

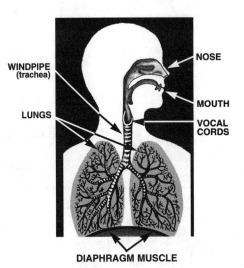

AIR SYSTEM FACTS

- Each lung weighs about one pound (.45 kg).
- A normal person takes in about 3000 gallons (113,400 l) of air each day.
- Air going into your lungs contains 21% oxygen and practically no carbon dioxide.
- Air going out of your lungs contains about 16% oxygen and 4% carbon dioxide.

Name _____

Measuring Your Lungs

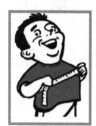

An adult man has room for about six quarts (5.7 l) of air in his lungs. An adult woman has room for five quarts (4.8 l). In normal breathing, you can only force about four quarts (3.8 l) of air in and out of your lungs.

Chest Expansion

1. Obtain a tape measure or a long string.

2. Breathe as deeply as possible. Measure the size of your chest. _____inches (cm)

3. Exhale as completely as possible. Measure the size of your chest. _____ inches (cm)

4. How much larger did your chest get when expanded? _____ inches (cm)

Measuring Your Lungs

How much air can you force out of your lungs? Here is a way to find out.

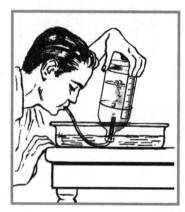

1. Obtain a half or one-gallon (1.9 or 3.8 l) clear plastic bottle, a large bowl and about two feet (.61 m) of rubber or plastic tubing.

2. Use rubber bands to mount a ruler on the bottle as shown.

3. Fill the bowl half full with water.

4. Fill the bottle *completely* with water.

5. Place your hand over the mouth of the bottle. Turn the bottle upside down in the bowl *below the water level*. Remove your hand. The water will stay in the bottle.

6. With the help of a friend, tilt the bottle and shove the hose a few inches (centimeters) inside the bottle.

7. Keep the bottle tilted so that the hose is not pinched.

8. Inhale as much air as you can, and use the hose to blow maximum air into the bottle. Use only *one breath*.

9. Measure the amount of inches (centimeters) of water your breath displaced. _____ inches (cm)

10. Wash off the hose, and repeat the breath experiment with friends.

Here is how you can get a rough idea of the quarts (liters) of air you expelled. Compare the inches (centimeters) of water removed to the total inches (centimeters) of the bottle. If you blew out half of the water in a one-gallon (3.8 l) bottle, your air volume was half a gallon or two quarts (1.9 l).

Name _____

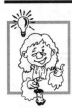

Measuring Your Breathing Rate

Your brain controls how fast you breathe. The carbon dioxide level in your blood triggers the brain. When you exercise vigorously, you produce more carbon dioxide. This signals the brain to have you breathe faster.

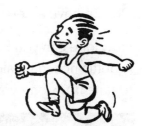

1. Sit still for two minutes.

2. While still sitting, count your breathing for one minute. Count inhaling and exhaling as one breath. _____ breaths

3. Now walk in place or walk around the room for two minutes. Count your breathing for one minute. _____ breaths

4. Now run in place or around the room for two minutes. Count your breathing rate for one minute. _____ breaths

5. Try these breathing rate experiments on some friends. How do their rates compare to yours?

COMPARING BREATHING RATES	
ANIMAL	**BREATHS PER MINUTE**
Newborn Child	55
Teenager	20
Adult	16
Giraffe	32
Horse	10
Rat	86
Rabbit	37

Name _____

Dr. Newton Wants You to Go Further

Do you have a pet? Try to count its normal (at rest) breathing rate.

How long can you hold your breath? A gray seal can hold its breath for 20 minutes. A bottle-nosed whale can hold its breath for almost two hours. Work with a friend to time how long you can hold your breath. _____ time

Caution: Don't exert yourself on this experiment. Don't try to go for a world's record.

You have learned that the diaphragm muscle helps you breathe. A lung model is shown below. Try to collect the materials needed to build it. You will need a one-hole rubber stopper, two rubber bands, plastic tubing, one large balloon, one small balloon and one common two-liter (1/2 gallon) plastic bottle.

Note: Your real body has two lungs. This model is simplified by showing only one lung.

1. Be **careful** in cutting the bottom off the plastic jar.

2. Move rubber diaphragm in or out to affect size of lung (balloon).

Dr. Newton wants you to know why people hiccup, yawn, cough or sneeze.

Hiccups: When you eat or drink too much, your stomach stretches and irritates the diaphragm. This causes the diaphragm to contract swiftly.

Yawns: When you are at rest, you breathe slowly. The lack of carbon dioxide triggers the brain to require an extra deep breath called a yawn.

Coughs or sneezes: Dirt irritates the windpipe or nose. Coughs and sneezes exhale large amounts of air suddenly to remove the irritating dirt.

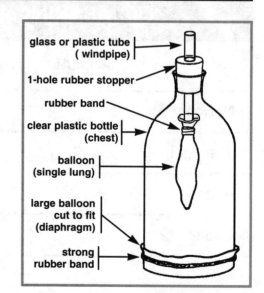

glass or plastic tube (windpipe)

1-hole rubber stopper

rubber band

clear plastic bottle (chest)

balloon (single lung)

large balloon cut to fit (diaphragm)

strong rubber band

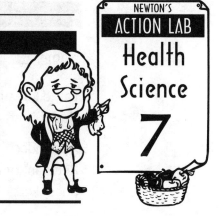

NEWTON'S
ACTION LAB
Health
Science
7

Digesting Your Food

Dr. Newton Wants You to Know

The digestive system passes food into the blood. Yet no one has ever found pizza, peas or hamburger in the blood. The job of the digestive system is to break these complex foods into simpler parts. Then these simpler parts can be dissolved into a liquid that passes into the blood. During your lifetime, your digestive system may handle over 60,000 pounds (27,000 kg) of food.

WHY YOUR BODY NEEDS FOOD

- For growth in size and strength.
- For repair of damaged or worn-out parts.
- For energy to provide warmth or motion.
- For maintaining the process of life.

How Your Digestive System Works

Your Mouth and Teeth
Teeth break up food while saliva softens food and starts to digest starch.

Esophagus
Passes food from mouth to stomach.

Stomach
Stomach muscles and digestive juices turn food into mush.

Small Intestine
Juices in intestine complete digestion and materials are passed to the blood.

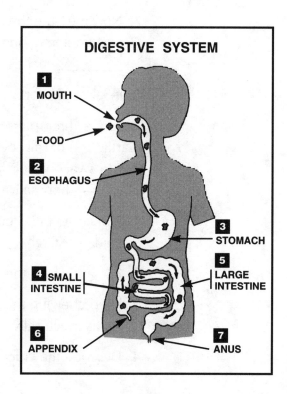

DIGESTIVE SYSTEM

1 MOUTH
FOOD
2 ESOPHAGUS
3 STOMACH
4 SMALL INTESTINE
5 LARGE INTESTINE
6 APPENDIX
7 ANUS

Name _____

Large Intestine

Water is absorbed back into blood and wastes are eliminated through the anus.

Appendix

Remnant of ancient man's second stomach. Needed when food was rougher and uncooked.

Anus

Where body wastes are eliminated.

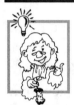

Investigating Digestion

How Long Is the Average Digestive System?

1. Obtain a long string and a yardstick.

2. Mark off 3" (7 cm) of string for your mouth.

3. Add 10" (25 cm) for your esophagus.

4. Add 6" (15 cm) for your stomach.

5. Add 15' (4.5 m) for your small intestine.

6. Add 5' (1.5 m) more for your large intestine.

7. Now measure the entire length of the string. How many feet (meters) and inches (centimeters) long is an average digestive system? _____ feet (m) _____ inches (cm)

Your Saliva at Work

There are three pairs of **salivary glands** around your mouth. They make about a quart (.95 l) of saliva each day. Saliva moistens your food so that it is slippery and easy to swallow. Saliva dissolves sugar and starts the digestion of starch. Find out for yourself how saliva can change starch into sugar.

1. Obtain an unsalted cracker. If not, use a regular cracker. Crackers are mainly made of starch.

2. Bite and chew the cracker. *Do not swallow it.* Describe the cracker's taste.

3. Keep chewing the cracker for at least one minute. Again, try not to swallow it. Let as much saliva as possible contact the starch in the cracker.

4. Describe the cracker's taste after the saliva has worked on it.

Name _____

Your Stomach Juices at Work

Your stomach is like a large muscular bag. The muscular stomach walls squeeze and break up food. Meanwhile, stomach juices act on the food. The result is that food leaving the stomach is mostly liquid.

1. Your stomach juices are acid. You can see how acids affect food by trying this experiment.

2. Place a raw egg into a glass or small jar.

3. Cover the egg with vinegar (an acid).

4. Wait 24 hours.

5. Describe how your eggshell looked and felt.

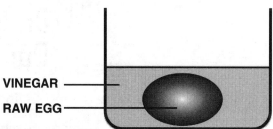

VINEGAR

RAW EGG

> The vinegar dissolved the calcium and other minerals that harden the shell. In much the same way, your stomach acids dissolve food.

Dr. Newton Wants You to Know More

PERISTALSIS IN THE ESOPHAGUS

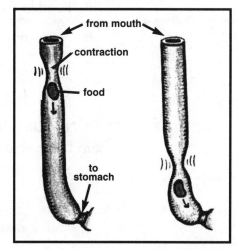

from mouth

contraction

food

to stomach

Your food does not just fall through your digestive system by gravity. Food is actually pushed through your system by a process called **peristalsis**. Peristalsis uses layers of muscle in your esophagus and intestines. These muscles relax and contract in a wave motion to pass food forward.

Dr. Newton wants you to demonstrate peristalsis for yourself. Here are some ways to imitate peristalsis.

1. Push a tennis ball through a sock. Form your fingers into a ring behind the ball. Work the ball forward in a peristaltic wave.

2. Do the same with a small bead and a straw or rubber tubing.

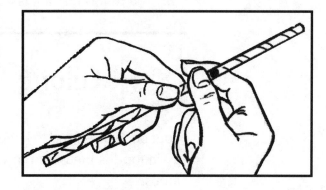

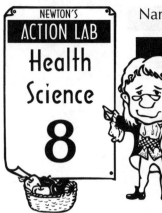

Name _____

Nutrition: You Are What You Eat

Dr. Newton Wants to Quiz You About Nutrition

Here is a test to find your nutrition I.Q. Answer true or false for each.

1. Being overweight is the most common physical problem among young people.

2. Overweight parents tend to have overweight children.

3. Overweight youngsters sometimes eat less than normal youngsters.

4. Bedtime snacks can cause indigestion, insomnia and nightmares.

5. The main ingredient in most foods is water.

6. People in cold climates need more calories than those in warm climates.

7. Food loses some of its nutrient value when cooked.

8. Fish is not a brain food.

9. Eating sugar does not cause diabetes.

10. Most vitamins are not stored in your body.

Dr. Newton wants you to take the "pinch the fat" test. Pinch the fat layer on the side of your body just below the rib. Have someone measure the fat layer between your fingers.

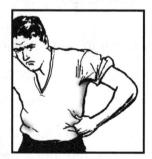

1. You're too chubby if it measures over 1" (2.5 cm).

2. You're normal if it is between $1/4$" to $1/2$" (.6 to 1.25 cm).

3. You're too thin if it is less than $1/4$" (.6 cm).

Calorie Counting

Your body uses food to keep warm and to provide energy to move about. The energy in food is measured in **calories**. Sugars, starches, fats and oils are high-calorie foods.

Name _____

CALORIES PER SERVING

cheese 100	fudge 115	pizza (cheese) 150
whole milk 150	jam 60	peanuts (1 cup [240 ml]) . .800
ice cream 270	bread (slice) 70	potato chips 115
butter 100	popcorn 25	

CALORIES USED PER HOUR

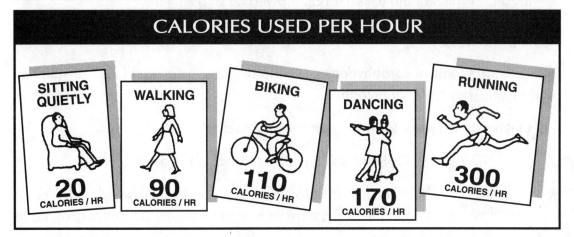

The calorie content of food is measured by burning the food and measuring energy output. Here is a simple method of understanding the calories in nuts.

1. Bend the end of a paper clip so that it forms a right angle.

2. Push the straight piece into a cork.

3. Place the peanut on the clip as shown.

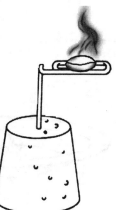

Caution: Do this over a sink and get an adult to supervise the burning.

4. Light the peanut from below. How long in seconds did it burn? _____ seconds

5. Try cashews or other nuts to see how long they burn.

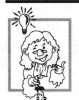

Food Tests

Testing for Fats and Oils

The simplest test for fats and oils involves rubbing food onto a paper bag. If fats or oils are present, the paper will change. It will become **translucent** which means that it will let more light through.

Name _____

1. Obtain a paper bag. Brown unglazed bags work best.

2. Cut the bag into 4" (10 cm) squares.

3. Rub various foods onto the center of the squares. Try peanuts, butter, cooking oil, olives, cheese, bananas, avocados or any convenient foods.

4. Hold the test paper up to a window or light. Describe how the fatty paper looked. Which of the tested foods showed fat or oils?

Testing for Starch

Starch is one form of **carbohydrates**. Carbohydrates include all kinds of starches and sugar. They are energy food.

1. Obtain some iodine from the medicine cabinet.

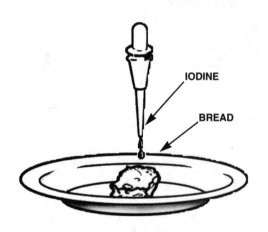

IODINE

BREAD

2. Obtain a shallow dish to work on to avoid a mess.

3. Place a drop of iodine on a piece of white bread. What color did the bread turn? Any starchy food will turn that color due to iodine.

4. Now collect potatoes, rice, apples, cheese and various foods. Which foods tested showed the color for starch?

5. Paper is often made with a starch binder. Try a drop of iodine on paper to find out if your paper contains starch.

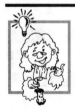

Dr. Newton Wants You to Read Food Labels

Some foods have **additives** to preserve, color or flavor them. Some additives actually improve your health. Salt often has iodine added that your body needs.

Check out some food labels. Reading food labels can be both interesting and useful. Use the form below to report additives. Simply place a check in the right category.

Food Tested	Sugar	Salt	Preservatives	Coloring	Flavoring
1.					
2.					
3.					
4.					
5.					
6.					

Name _____

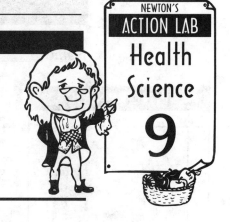

ACTION LAB
Health
Science
9

Your Thin Skin

Dr. Newton Wants You to Know

Your skin is the largest organ of your body. An adult skin can weigh nine pounds (4 kg) and be over 20 square feet (1.8 sq. m) in area.

WHAT YOUR SKIN DOES FOR YOU

- It is a barrier that protects your body from disease and injury.
- It receives information from the environment through nerves that respond to pressure, pain, heat or cold.
- It helps control your body temperature by evaporation from your sweat glands.
- It helps eliminate your body's waste material.

Study the cross section of skin shown at the right. The **epidermis** is the outer skin layer. Its top has dead and dying cells that your body is constantly shedding. The bottom of the epidermis is made of living, active cells.

The **dermis** is the portion of the skin below the epidermis. It makes new skin cells to replace the worn-out cells. It contains nerves, muscle and a blood supply. The dermis also contains glands that oil your skin and make you sweat.

The bottom skin layer contains mainly fat. This cushions your skin and attaches to your muscle.

Your nails are part of your skin. They are made of dead cells so cutting them doesn't hurt. Nails protect your sensitive fingers and toes. You can measure how fast your nails grow.

Observe the white "half-moon" at the base of your nails. Nails grow from here and are pushed outward.

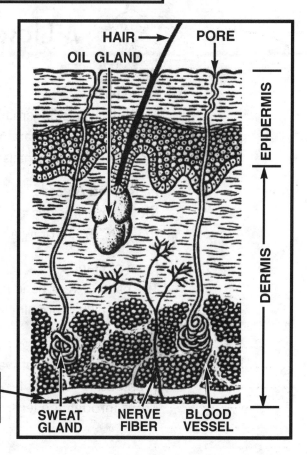

HAIR → PORE
OIL GLAND
EPIDERMIS
DERMIS
FATTY LAYER
SWEAT GLAND   NERVE FIBER   BLOOD VESSEL

TLC10143 Copyright © Teaching & Learning Company, Carthage, IL 62321-0010

Name _____

FINGERNAIL

tip

base

half-moon

1. Measure the nail length of your middle finger as shown.

2. Measure as **exactly** as you can to the nearest $1/16$" (.16 cm). _____ inches (cm)

3. Nails grow very slowly. Don't cut the middle fingernail and measure it again in two weeks. _____ inches (cm)

How much did your nail grow in two weeks? _____

Be brave and try again after a month.

SKIN FACTS

- Your entire skin can wear away and be replaced every year.
- Fingernails grow three times faster than toenails.
- Your skin color is due to a substance called melanin.
- Heredity and sun rays determine your skin color.
- Skin varies in thickness. It is thinnest over your eyes and the thickest on the soles of your feet.

A Close Look at Your Skin

Fingernails
Look at various fingernails and compare their color markings. What size and shape are the hardened margins of skin around the nails, called *cuticles*? Notice the half-moon base of your nails. Sketch your own and a friend's fingernails.

Pigmented Areas
Moles and freckles are concentrated areas of a dark brown-red pigment called *melanin*. Try to draw an exact outline of a few pigmented areas.

Palm of Hand
The palm of your hand has a large number of sweat glands. Observe that the sweat glands make your palm look more "waxy" than the rest of your skin.

Water on Wrist
Place a few drops of water on your wrist. How does your skin feel as the water evaporates? That is how your body cools itself by sweating. Observe the water drops through the lens. Describe the appearance of the water on your skin.

Name _____

Hair Differences
Carefully cut a long hair from yourself and two friends. Line them up on a sheet of white paper. Compare the three hairs for differences in thickness, curl, color and transparency.

Skin Freedom
In the spirit of health science, you are encouraged to use your lens to further explore your epidermis.

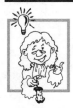

Your Unique Fingerprints

Your fingers have patterns on them that are unique to you. They are formed by bumps and ridges on your dermis that projects through the epidermis. These fingerprint patterns remain the same for your entire life.

Fingerprints can be used to identify criminals or lost children. You would have to fingerprint billions of people before finding two that are alike. Even identical twins do not have the same fingerprints.

1. Obtain a stamp pad and white paper.

2. Roll your thumb from left to right *lightly* over the ink pad.

3. Roll your inked thumb from left to right over the white paper.

4. Repeat for your other four fingers.

Compare your fingerprints to the three basic fingerprint patterns shown. Remember that there are many variations of these basic prints. It might help to use a lens. Fingerprint some friends and compare them to yours.

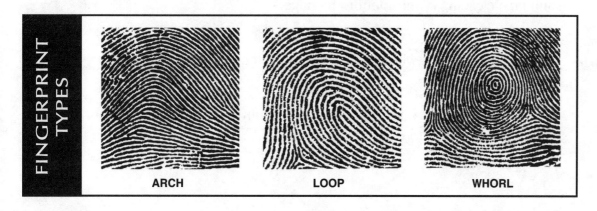

FINGERPRINT TYPES

ARCH   LOOP   WHORL

Name _____

Dr. Newton Answers Some Skin Questions

How Many Hairs Are There on Your Head?

The average scalp has about 100,000 hairs. The actual count may depend on your age, whether you are male or female or whether your hair is coarse or fine.

The easy way to count scalp hairs is to pull one hair from a person's scalp and declare that they have one less than before. Here is a more practical but very imperfect way to obtain a hair count.

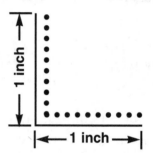

1. Use a ruler to roughly count the hairs along 1" (2.5 cm) of scalp. _____ hairs

2. Now make a 1" (2.5 cm) hair count at right angles to the other inch (cm). ____ hairs

3. Multiply the two hair counts to get a rough idea of the number of hairs per square inch (sq. cm). For example, you might have a 22 by 24 count for a square inch (sq. cm) total of 550 hairs. _____ hairs per square inch (sq. cm)

You're still not done. You have to estimate the total square inches (sq. cm) on your scalp. This can be done in many ways, but let's save you the trouble. Young people might have approximately 70 square inches (440 sq. cm) of scalp. An adult might have 80 square inches (500 sq. cm).

4. Multiply your square inch (sq. cm) count by 70 (440 sq. cm). Your estimated total hair count is _____ hairs.

What Causes Acne?
The surface openings of your oil glands get filled with oil and dirt. That's why constant face cleaning is important to teenagers.

What Causes Warts?
Warts are caused by a virus that commonly affects children.

What Causes Freckles?
Freckles are harmless concentrations of melanin that are found on your face and arms. Sunlight tends to darken your freckles.

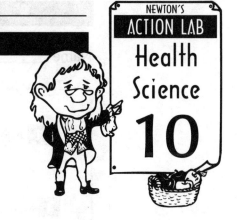

You Are Just a Bag of Bones

Dr. Newton Wants You to Know

Your body is shaped, held erect and protected by your bones. Muscles acting on your bones can move you in almost any direction.

Your bones are alive. They require food to grow, repair themselves and manufacture blood cells. They especially need calcium, phosphorus and other minerals to grow strong.

At birth, you have almost 300 bones in your body. These bones are soft and flexible. As you grow older, your bones harden and some fuse together. An adult only has about 206 bones.

Where Your Bones Are

Skull: 29 bones including 3 tiny ear bones

Spine: 26 bones

Breastbone and Ribs: 25 bones

Shoulders, Arms and Hands: 64 bones

Pelvis, Legs and Feet: 62 bones

Your Bones Are Latin

Dr. Newton learned to be a doctor in medical school. Body parts in medical schools are given Latin names. These are the same names used by doctors in all countries no matter what language is spoken.

The chart on page 36 has your bones identified in Latin and numbered. Unscramble the words to the right of the chart to find out their common names in English.

Name _____

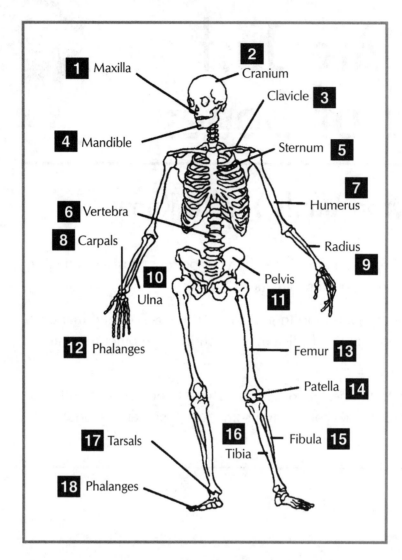

Labels in diagram:
1 Maxilla
2 Cranium
3 Clavicle
4 Mandible
5 Sternum
6 Vertebra
7 Humerus
8 Carpals
9 Radius
10 Ulna
11 Pelvis
12 Phalanges
13 Femur
14 Patella
15 Fibula
16 Tibia
17 Tarsals
18 Phalanges

1. **UPPER WAJBONE**
2. **LLUSK**
3. **NCOBARLLOE**
4. **LOWER AJW BONE**
5. **BEEAOSTRBN**
6. **PSINE**
7. **UPPER RAM BONE**
8. **RISTW**
9. **LOWER RAM BONE**
10. **LOWER RAM BONE**
11. **PIH BONE**
12. **FIGNESR**
13. **THGHI**
14. **NEEKPAC**
15. **SIHN BONES**
16. **SIHN BONES**
17. **AKLEN**
18. **SEOT**

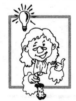

Using a Bone to Measure Your Height

Each bone in your body grows in proportion to the rest of your bones. In this activity you are going to measure the length of your radius. The radius is one of the two bones in your lower arm. You can use this one bone measurement to try to estimate your total height.

RADIUS
WRIST
ELBOW

1. Rest your elbow on a desk with your lower arm straight up at 90°.

2. Measure in inches (centimeters) from your elbow to your wrist. _____ inches (cm). This is approximately the length of your radius.

36

Name _____

3. Compute your estimated height using the formulas below.

Boys	**Girls**
Your Height = 3R + 34	Your Height = 3R + 33

Example: *A boy has a 9" (23 cm) radius. His estimated height will be*

3 x 9 + 34 = 27 + 34 = 61 inches = 5 feet 1 inch (155 cm)

What is your estimated height using your radius? _____ inches (cm)

What is your real measured height? _____ inches (cm)

How many inches (cm) off were you? _____ inches (cm)

4. Try measuring other people using this method. Don't expect perfect answers. Everybody grows differently.

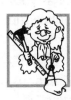

Dr. Newton Can Bend Your Bones

Drink your milk and eat your vegetables. These foods contain the calcium and other minerals you need for strong bones.

Without minerals, your rigid bones would be soft and flexible. You can discover this by soaking chicken bones in vinegar. Vinegar is an acid that removes minerals.

1. Find two similar, long chicken bones.

2. Clean them thoroughly. Leave no meat on the bones.

3. Place one in an empty jar. Scientists call this bone a **control**. You will use it to compare with the vinegar bone.

4. Place the other bone in a jar. Cover the bone with vinegar and wait five days.

5. After five days, wash the vinegar bone thoroughly.

6. Describe the differences between the vinegar and the control bones.

Be good to your bones. Eat mineral foods.

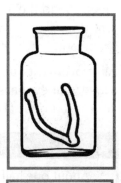

CONTROL (no vinegar)

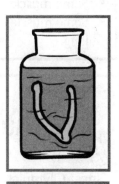

VINEGAR

Name _____

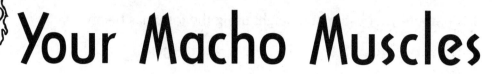

Your Macho Muscles

Dr. Newton Wants You to Know

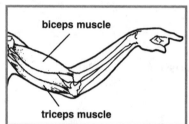

biceps muscle

triceps muscle

Your muscles work in pairs. One muscle pulls a bone one way. A partner muscle pulls on the bone the opposite way. The pulling muscle gets shorter. The relaxed muscle gets longer. You can feel this for yourself on your upper arm.

Place your left hand on the top muscle of your right upper arm. You are touching a muscle called the **biceps**. Make a tight fist and bring the fist toward your shoulder. Your biceps will shorten and become harder as your arm is raised. Unclench your fist, and stretch your arm out in front of you. Notice the change in the size, shape and hardness of your biceps.

Now place your left hand *under* your upper arm. You are touching a muscle called the **triceps**. The triceps and biceps are paired muscles that pull in opposite directions. Biceps bend the arm while triceps straighten the arm. Make a tight fist, and move your arm toward and away from your shoulder. You can feel your triceps changing in size, shape and hardness.

All movements of your body use at least two muscles working against each other. Move your eyeballs up and down and sideways. Six muscles control these movements. Your face needs about 150 of your body's 600 muscles to talk, smile or cry.

MUSCLE FACTS

- About one-half of a man's weight is muscle.
- About one-third of a woman's weight is muscle.
- Some muscles are 12" (30 cm) long.
- Some muscles are less than 1" (2.5 cm) long.
- The biggest muscles are in your buttocks. They help you jump.
- The smallest muscles are in your ear.
- About 200 muscles work together when you walk.

Muscle Strength

Finger Olympics

Test your finger muscles by competing with a friend.

Name _____

1. Make a fist, and place your arm firmly on a table.

2. Lock your fingers, as shown, and pull. Both arms should still rest on the table.

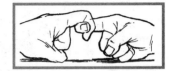

3. The first to let go has the weakest finger muscles.

4. Challenge other people to the Finger Olympics.

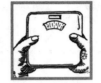

Your Muscles Versus a Bathroom Scale

Challenge your friends to a bathroom scale competition.

1. Squeeze the bathroom scale with both hands as shown in the drawing. How many pounds (kilograms) did your fingers squeeze? _____ pounds (kg)

2. Sit on a chair with the scale against a wall as shown in the drawing.

3. Use your foot muscles to obtain the highest reading you can. How many pounds (kilograms) did your foot push? _____ pounds (kg)

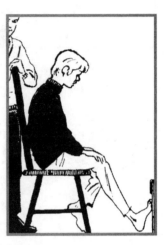

Try different ways of using a bathroom scale to measure other muscles. You could test head and neck muscles, your big toe muscles, your biceps.

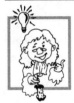

Muscle Fatigue

Exercise helps your muscles become stronger. Sometimes overworked muscles suddenly tighten up and become painful. This is called a **cramp**. More often, overworked muscles become weary and slow down. This is called **fatigue**. Muscles that suffer from fatigue have run out of the oxygen and food they need. They require a rest to obtain more oxygen and food and to get rid of wastes.

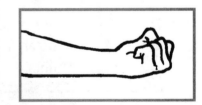

You can check muscle fatigue for yourself with these simple exercises. You will need a watch or wall clock with a second hand.

1. Hold your right arm straight out in front of you.

2. Open and close your fist as rapidly as you can. Count the number of fist closures in 30 seconds. _____

3. Rest **only** 15 seconds.

4. Repeat the fist closures for another 30 seconds. Your poor fist suffered from fatigue.

5. How many times was it able to open and close the second time? _____

6. How many less fist closures were you able to do while fatigued? _____

Name _____

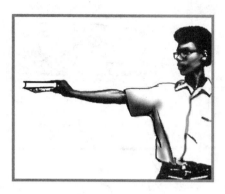

Now let's try to fatigue your bulging biceps.

1. Hold a book in your hand.

2. Raise your arm from straight down at your side to straight out 90° in front of you.

3. Count the number of times you can do this in 30 seconds. _____

4. Rest **only** 15 seconds.

5. Again, count the number of times your fatigued biceps raised the book in 30 seconds. _____

Compare the two trials.

There are other muscles in your body. Pick your favorite muscles, and design a 30-second fatigue exercise for them.

Dr. Newton Wants You to Learn More About Muscles

Your Unsteady Muscles

Some muscles in your body are controlled by you. Some muscles are called **involuntary** because you really do not control them. Eyelid muscles are mainly involuntary. You cannot keep your eyes from blinking.

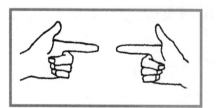

1. Stare ahead and try not to blink.

2. Bring two of your fingers close but not touching. (See the drawing.)

3. Try to keep your fingers perfectly steady without moving them at all.

4. Describe your results.

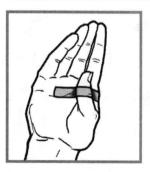

Your Wonderful Thumb

Observe your thumb. Unlike most other animals, your thumb can bend into your other fingers. Your thumb and its muscles help you do many things. Find out how important your thumb is by taping your right thumb to the palm of your hand. Then try to use your hand for normal activities. What are some of the things your taped hand couldn't do?

Name _____

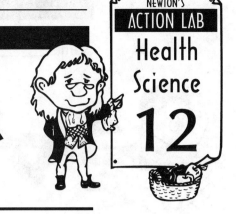

Your Senses at Work

Dr. Newton Wants You to Know

Your five senses help you connect to the world around you. The environment keeps sending you messages through your senses of sight, hearing, smell, taste and touch.

Your senses help you enjoy the sight and smell of flowers, the song of birds and the taste of chocolate. They can also warn you of danger in your environment such as an on-coming car or a polluted pond.

This section will investigate your sense of touch and the chemical senses of your tongue and nose.

Enter the World of the Deaf and Blind

Helen Keller was a famous American woman. When she was two, an illness left her both deaf and blind. She contacted the world around her by her sense of touch.

She learned to read **braille**. This is a system using raised dots on paper. By touching lips, she was able to understand what people were saying.

Helen Keller improved her sense of touch with practice. Can you improve your sense of touch with practice?

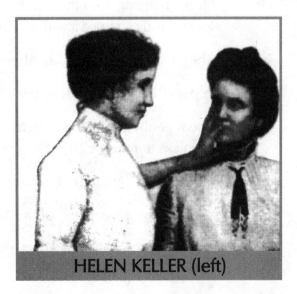

HELEN KELLER (left)

Name _____

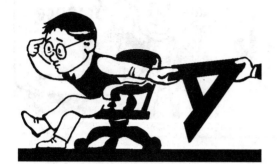

Alphabet Identification

1. Obtain eight cardboard or plastic alphabet letters. Cut out your own if necessary. Children's blocks with raised alphabet letters work fine.

2. Seat a friend. Have the friend look forward while you pass all eight letters to him or her from behind.

3. How many of the eight letters did your friend identify by touch alone? _____

4. Switch places. How many did you identify? _____

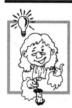

Your Sense of Touch

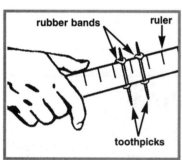

Pressure Nerves

Your skin has almost five million nerve endings. There are around 250,000 nerve endings on your body that respond to pressure. Even with that many, you are often not sure whether you are being touched by one or two objects.

Study the gadget on the left. It will let you experiment with your sense of touch. You can build it with toothpicks, a ruler and two small rubber bands.

1. Adjust the toothpicks so they are about ¹/₂" (1.25 cm) apart.

2. Work in pairs. Have the person being tested close their eyes.

3. Touch them gently on the back of the arm 10 times. Touch them with one or two toothpicks at random.

4. How many of the 10 random touches did they guess correctly? _____

5. Reverse positions. How many of the 10 touches did you recognize? _____

6. Try the touch test on your wrist, back of your neck, palm of your hand, index finger or "?".

Some areas of your skin have the pressure nerves very close. Some areas have the pressure nerves far apart. What touch areas were you most successful in guessing correctly?

Name _____

Temperature Nerves

Your skin has 150,000 nerves that respond to cold. Only 16,000 respond to heat. Let's try to fool your temperature nerves.

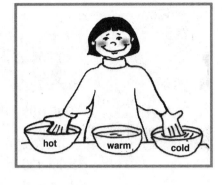

1. Obtain three similar bowls or jars.

2. Fill one with hot water. **Caution!** Not too hot!

3. Fill one with cold water.

4. Fill one with lukewarm water.

5. Line them up as shown. Place one hand in the hot and one in the cold water.

6. Wait one full minute.

7. **Quickly** place **both** hands in the lukewarm water. Describe the sensation.

Your Sense of Taste

Your taste sense is sometimes called a **chemical** sense. You only taste things because chemicals leave the food and affect your taste nerves.

Look at your tongue in a mirror. You will be able to see bumps. Each bump has between 100 and 200 taste buds.

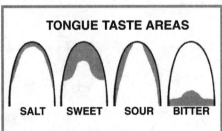

TONGUE TASTE AREAS

SALT SWEET SOUR BITTER

Study the tongue maps on the right. They show the areas of the tongue that are responsible for salty, sweet, sour and bitter tastes. Now try to check the taste areas on someone's tongue.

1. Obtain **clean** toothpicks, sugar water, salt water, a bit of vinegar in water for sour and a baby aspirin dissolved in water for the bitter taste.

2. Use a **clean** toothpick for each test.

3. Try sugar water on all four taste areas. Describe your results.

4. Try salt water on all four taste areas. Describe your results.

5. Try vinegar water (sour) on all four taste areas. Describe your results.

6. Try aspirin water (bitter) on all four taste areas. Describe your results.

7. Try bits of various **clean** foods on all four taste areas. Describe your results.

What foods did you have difficulty recognizing by taste?

Name _____

Your Sense of Smell

Your smell nerves are high up in your nose. Smelling, like tasting, depends upon chemicals in the air to affect the nerve endings.

Collect five to 10 different odors. Blindfold your friends, and see if they can identify the odors. Try onion, pickle, vinegar, flowers, lemon or "?".

Your taste ability often depends on your sense of smell.

1. Cut up some small cubes of raw potato, apple, onion, pickle or "?".

2. Blindfold your friends and have them hold their nose.

3. Let them chew on each food cube. **Think sanitation.**

Which food cubes were they able to identify by taste without using their sense of smell?

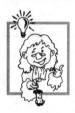

Dr. Newton's Sensory Fun

Don't hurt yourself on this experiment. Strike your elbow **gently** on a table. There is an *ulnar* nerve at your elbow that often gives you combined sensations of pain, tingling, cold or warm.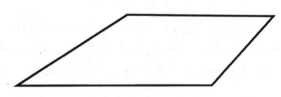
That's why your elbow is sometimes called your "funny" bone.

Study the drawing on the right. Do you think that you could place a nickel, penny or dime inside the drawing without touching a line? Try it.

SENSE FACTS

- Dogs have a sense of smell 100 times better than humans.
- You lose some your sense of smell as you grow older.
- You can see better in dim light by **not** staring at an object. Let your eyes flick from the right to the left of the object.

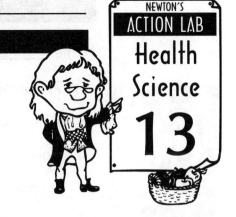

Investigating Your Eyes

Dr. Newton Wants You to Know

The eye is the most important of your five senses. Still, your eye can be fooled easily. Study the picture to the right carefully. There are two different pictures.

Light enters your eye through a thin clear tissue called the **cornea**. Behind the cornea is the colored part of your eye called the **iris**. The dark center of the iris is actually an opening called the **pupil**. The iris muscles adjust the pupil size to control the amount of light that is allowed to enter.

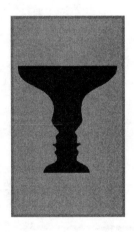

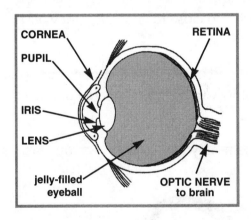

Behind the pupil is the **lens**. Unlike lenses in eyeglasses, your eye has muscles that can change the shape of the lens. You need to change the shape to focus on near or far objects.

The light focused by the lens falls on the **retina** in the back of your eyeball. The retina contains nerve endings that are sensitive to light. The nerves run through the optic nerve to the brain which interprets what you see.

Mirror Your Eyes

Observing Your Eyes

Use a mirror on your own eyes or work with a partner to observe each other. Identify all the front parts of the eye in the drawing. You should observe the dark pupil and the colored iris. See if the white part of your eye has blood vessels showing. Try to see the tiny hole that drains tears in the nose corner of the eye. Can you make a simple sketch of what you see?

Name _____

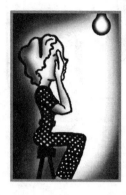

Your Pupils at Work

The iris of your eye adjusts the pupil opening in response to the quantity of light.

1. Work with a partner.

2. Sit on a chair facing an **indoor** light source. **Caution!** Do not look at the sun.

3. Close your eyes for one full minute while still facing the light source.

4. Open your eyes and have your partner observe the pupil change. What happened to your pupils as the light hit your eyes?

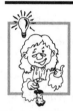

More Complicated Eye Tests

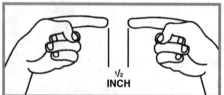

Two-Eyed Vision

Normally your two eyes work together as a team to focus on objects. When you bring objects too close to your eyes, they have difficulty working together.

Place your two index fingers ¹/₂" (1.25 cm) apart and about 10" (25 cm) in front of your eyes. Keep them ¹/₂" (1.25 cm) apart and slowly bring them toward your face. What do you see between the fingers?

Note the arrow and target below. Stare at them as you slowly bring your face toward them. What appeared to happen?

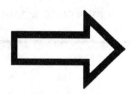 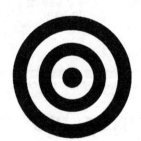

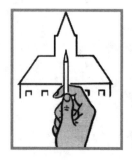

Your Dominant Eye

Most people have one eye that dominates the other. Here's a way to find out which of your eyes dominates.

Line up your finger with a distant object using **both** eyes. Now close first the left and then the right eye. With your dominant eye (usually the right), the finger and the distant object remain lined up. With your weak eye, they jump out of line.

Name _____

Astigmatism Test

Sometimes the transparent cornea that covers your eye is not perfectly formed. This is called **astigmatism**.

Look at the lined wheel picture to the right. If your cornea is not perfect, some of the lines will appear blurred at normal reading distance.

Please don't take this test too seriously. Only an eye doctor with a real chart can tell if you have a problem.

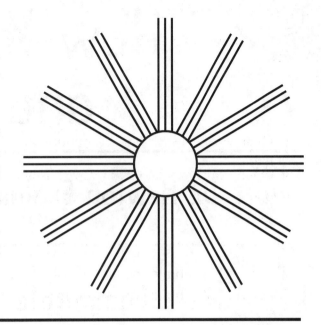

Dr. Newton's Eye Specials

1. Look closely at the back of a penny. You should be able to see Lincoln's face inside the Lincoln Memorial.

2. Go outside at night, and identify the Big Dipper. The second star from the end of the handle is really two stars.

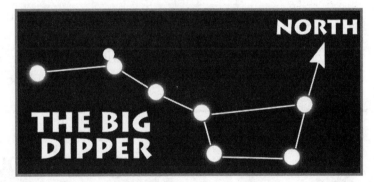

EYELID FACTS

- Blinking helps your salty antiseptic tears clean your eyes.
- Your eyelids are controlled by your fastest body muscles.
- You can blink up to five times a second.
- You normally blink every two to 12 seconds.
- The average person blinks 20,000 times every day.

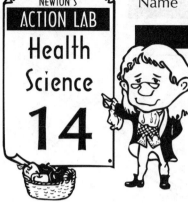
How You Hear and Talk

Dr. Newton Explains Your Ear

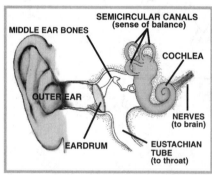

SEMICIRCULAR CANALS
(sense of balance)

MIDDLE EAR BONES

COCHLEA

OUTER EAR

NERVES
(to brain)

EARDRUM

EUSTACHIAN
TUBE
(to throat)

All sound is due to vibration. When you talk, your vocal cords vibrate the air. Air vibrations from sounds move into your ear and vibrate your eardrum.

This vibrates three tiny bones called the **hammer**, **anvil** and **stirrup**.

The vibrating bones cause vibrations inside the **cochlea**. This is a snail-like structure filled with fluids and nerve endings. The nerve endings connect to the brain which interprets the sounds you hear.

The **semicircular canals** above your inner ear are responsible for your sense of balance. The **eustachian tube** connects the middle ear to your throat. It serves to equalize air pressure inside and outside your ear. You may have felt the pain of unequal pressure in your ear while flying in an airplane.

Experimenting with Your Vocal Cords

Feeling Your Vocal Cords

Feel the lump on your throat that is called the Adam's apple. It is your voice box and contains the two thin muscles of your vocal cords. Hum loudly as you touch your vocal cords. You will feel them vibrating to make sound.

Balloon Vocal Cords

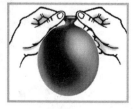

Blow up a balloon to the size of your head. Hold each side of the balloon with your thumb and forefingers as shown. Stretch the mouth of the balloon as the air escapes to make high and low sounds. Your vocal cords also stretch to make different sounds.

Name _____

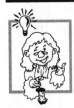

Testing Your Ears

How Far Can You Hear?

Work with others to measure the distance at which you can no longer hear a standard sound. The standard sound could be any of the below:

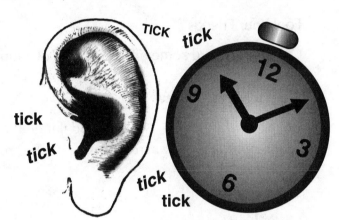

- a ticking watch
- a rubber band around a box
- a clicking ballpoint pen
- a marble dropped into a can
- a radio set at a low level
- a sound maker of your own invention

1. Measure and record the distance at which people stop hearing the standard sound.

   Person 1 _____ feet (m)   Person 2 _____ feet (m)   Person 3 _____ feet (m)

2. Try checking your friends, parents and grandparents to find if age affects hearing distance ability.

It Takes Two Ears to Determine Sound Direction

Use your standard sound to check your ability to identify the direction of sound.

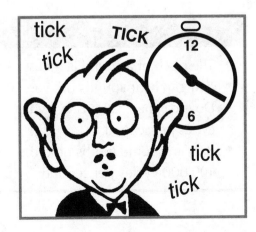

1. Close your eyes. Have a friend make a sound from various locations around you. Can you point to the sound's correct direction?

2. Close your eyes again.

Name _____

3. **Cover one ear** with your hand so that no sound can enter.

4. Have a friend again make sounds from various directions. Could you detect sound better with one or two ears?

Dr. Newton's Favorite Sound Ideas

Fool Your Friends

Collect or record some different kinds of sounds. Can your friends identify them?

Make a Musical Straw

Cut a straw as shown. Moisten and flatten the cut end. Place the **entire** cut end in your mouth and blow across it. Be patient. You may have to try different straws or different cuts.

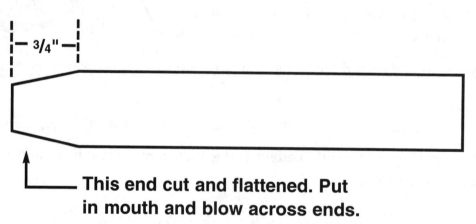

|– 3/4" –|

This end cut and flattened. Put in mouth and blow across ends.

EAR FACTS

- The pitch of a sound is measured in cycles per second.
- You can hear sounds between 15 and 20,000 cycles per second.
- Dogs can hear sounds that you can't. They can hear sounds as high as 50,000 cycles per second.
- Bats and some moths hold the hearing record. They can hear sounds up to 100,000 cycles per second.

50

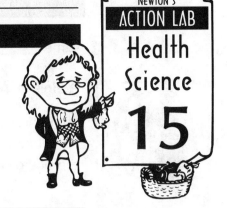

NEWTON'S
ACTION LAB
Health Science
15

Your Brain at Work

Dr. Newton Wants You to Know

Your brain, spinal cord and nerves make up your nervous system. The brain interprets messages from your environment. The messages are transmitted through the nerves and spinal cord to the brain.

Your brain weighs about three pounds (1.4 kg). It is shaped like a giant walnut. If the brain were unfolded, it would cover almost a square yard (sq. m).

Your brain has three main areas. Each has a job to do. The **cerebrum** is the largest part. Different areas in your cerebrum are responsible for such things as memory, speech and motion.

Messages are carried to and from your brain by cells called **neurons**. Neurons can be very short or very long. They carry messages both chemically and electrically.

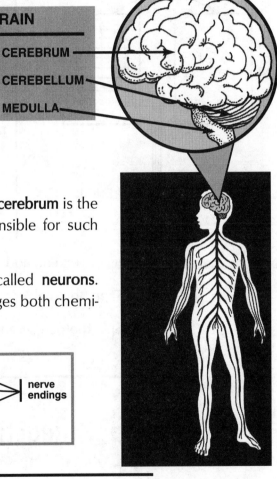

BRAIN
- CEREBRUM
- CEREBELLUM
- MEDULLA

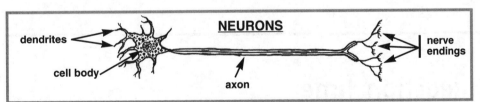

NEURONS

dendrites

cell body

axon

nerve endings

Fooling Your Brain

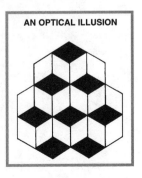

AN OPTICAL ILLUSION

Your brain has more power than an expensive computer. Yet, it can be fooled easily.

Optical Illusion

Observe the optical illusion on the right. Do you see six or seven cubes?

Name _____

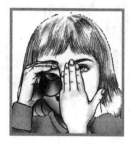

A Hole in Your Hand

Look through a toilet paper roll with your right eye. Bring the side of your other hand to the center of the roll. View with **both eyes** open. Do you see a "hole" in the side of your hand?

How Movies Fool Your Brain

Movies are an optical illusion. They take advantage of the fact that when your eyes see over 20 pictures a second, your brain blends them into motion. A cowboy chasing a cow in a movie is really a series of still pictures that your brain blends into motion.

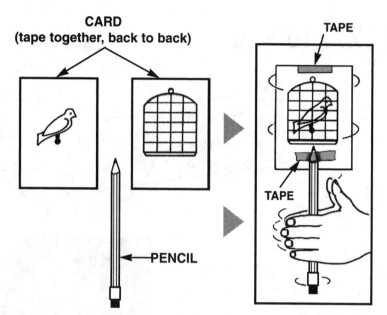

CARD
(tape together, back to back)

←PENCIL

TAPE

TAPE

1. Cut a 3" x 5" (8 x 13 cm) card in half.

2. Draw a bird with **sharp dark** lines on one half of the card.

3. Draw a larger bird cage with **sharp dark** lines on the other half.

4. If convenient, add color lines to your drawings.

5. Tape both halves to a pencil.

6. Spin the pencil **rapidly** between your hands as shown. What do you observe?

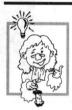

Reaction Time

You see a ball coming toward you. You blink and pull away. Your eyes signaled your brain. Your brain signaled your muscles to react. Brains, nerves and muscles all must work together.

Card Game Reaction Time

1. Shuffle a full deck of cards.

2. Time how many seconds it takes you to remove all 13 spades and line them up ace through king. _____ total seconds

52

Name _____

3. Reshuffle all the cards and practice a few times.

4. After some practice, reshuffle the cards and time yourself again. _____ seconds

Did you improve with practice? Most people improve their reaction time with practice.

Dropped Ruler Reaction Time

1. Obtain a ruler. Place your hand on a table so that your thumb and index finger extend over the table.

2. Have a friend hold the zero end of the ruler between your thumb and index finger.

3. Without warning, your friend will drop the ruler. Use your thumb and index finger to grab the falling ruler. Practice a few times. Did you get better or worse with practice?

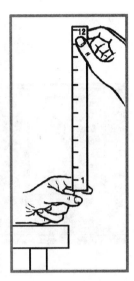

Here's a scale to rate your reaction time.

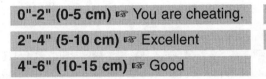

0"-2" (0-5 cm) ☞ You are cheating.	**6"-8" (15-20 cm)** ☞ Fair
2"-4" (5-10 cm) ☞ Excellent	**8"-12" (20-30 cm)** ☞ You need help!
4"-6" (10-15 cm) ☞ Good	

Dr. Newton Wants You to Stretch Your Imagination

Human beings have very advanced brains. The brain can do more than respond to signals from the environment. It can also remember and imagine.

Put your brain to the imagination test. Try to imagine something unreal.

1. Close your eyes and try to imagine a green horse running around on white grass.

2. Imagine yourself flying like a bird and observing the Earth.

3. Imagine yourself as a 2" (5 cm) person trying to survive outdoors.

BRAIN FACTS

- The brain is only 2% of your body weight. Yet it uses up 20% of your energy.
- Babies are born with about 14 billion neurons. Very few new ones are added as you grow.
- Nerve impulse can travel at speeds up to 400 feet (120 m) per second. Messages can cross from one nerve to another in less than $1/10,000$ of a second.

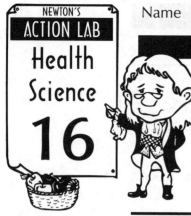

Name _____

Investigating Alcohol

Dr. Newton Wants You to Know

Drinking alcohol affects the brain rapidly. Alcohol is considered a chemical that depresses the brain.

People under the influence of alcohol act like they have gone without sleep for a long time. Senses are deadened, and the brain's control over body movement and reaction time is lessened. Memory, reflexes, accuracy, speed, learning and coordination are all affected.

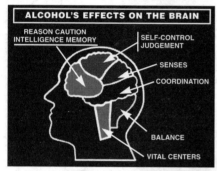

ALCOHOL'S EFFECTS ON THE BRAIN

REASON CAUTION
INTELLIGENCE MEMORY
SELF-CONTROL
JUDGEMENT
SENSES
COORDINATION
BALANCE
VITAL CENTERS

ALCOHOL FACTS

- One in four American families have alcohol-related problems.
- Almost half of all driving deaths involve alcoholic drinks.
- Forty percent of teenagers who drop out of school have alcohol problems.
- Half of police arrests involving murder and serious assaults are alcohol related.

Alcohol Versus Water

If you were forced to choose between alcohol and water, you would have no trouble making up your mind which is best. Life on Earth is based upon water, not alcohol. Your body needs and is made of water. Alcohol has no place inside your body.

Alcohol has a large variety of unique qualities which makes it valuable above and beyond its use as a beverage. Alcohol can be used as a disinfectant, cleaning fluid, antifreeze, anesthetic, explosive and preservative. It can be used in the manufacture of perfumes, medicines, dyes, paints, film, textiles, rubber and plastics.

1. Do all experiments using rubbing alcohol. **Caution!** Rubbing alcohol is a **poison** and should *never* enter your body.

2. Place some alcohol on one wrist. Place some water on the other wrist. Which seems colder? _____ This is due to alcohol evaporating faster.

54

Name _____

3. Smell the alcohol. Smell the water. Describe the difference.

4. Tear off two pieces of bread about 1" (2.5 cm) square. Do not use the crust.

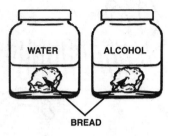

5. Place each square in a different jar. Just barely cover one with water. Just barely cover the other with alcohol.

6. Wait two minutes. Remove both squares. Let them dry a while and feel them.

7. Describe the differences. Alcohol actually removes water from the bread to dehydrate it.

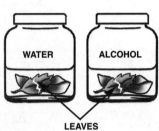

8. Tear up some leaves into very small pieces.

9. Place half the leaves in a small jar, and cover it with water.

10. Place the rest of the leaves in a similar jar, and cover it with rubbing alcohol.

11. Cover the jars and shake vigorously.

12. Wait about 30 minutes.

13. Compare both jars. The green material in leaves is a substance called chlorophyll. Is water or alcohol a better solvent of chlorophyll?

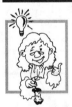

Pseudodrunk Activity

You are going to become **pseudodrunk** (false drunk) in this activity. Methods other than drinking alcohol will be used to temporarily muddle your brain and slow your reaction time. You will contrast your ability to perform certain tasks while you are sober and while you are pseudodrunk.

All the reaction tests will compare your normal response to your pseudo-drunk response. Only one person is to get "drunk" at a time. For maximum effect, take the tests **immediately** after making yourself pseudodrunk.

Here's how to get psuedodrunk. Sit in a chair and hold on to the seat. Lower your head and shake it sideways vigorously for 15 seconds.

Caution: Have a few friends surround you when you get psuedodrunk to avoid falling. Skip this activity if dizziness bothers you.

Name _____

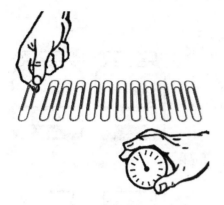

1. Obtain 12 paper clips and a watch with a second hand.

2. Line up the 12 paper clips in a row.

3. Attach as many together in a line as you can in 15 seconds.

4. How many did you attach in 15 seconds? _____

5. Line up 12 more paper clips.

6. Now review the cautions of spinning to become pseudodrunk. Remember to have others watch you.

7. Get psuedodrunk, and **immediately** try to attach as many paper clips as you can in 15 seconds.

8. How many did you attach while pseudodrunk in 15 seconds? _____ Was your coordination and speed better or worse while psuedodrunk?

9. Repeat the paper clip activity using your friends.

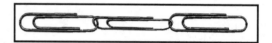

You can also check pseudodrunk reactions using playing cards. Pull out the ace to king of spades. Shuffle them. Repeat the pseudodrunk test by seeing how many seconds it takes to line up the cards from ace to king. It is even more challenging to require the experimenter to line up the cards with **only one hand**.

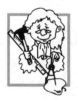

Dr. Newton Wants You to Know About Alcoholics Anonymous

Alcoholics Anonymous is an organization also known as AA. Their goal is to help members avoid the problems and temptations of alcohol. There is even a teen AA. For further information, you may contact the organization at this address: Alcoholics Anonymous, Box 459, Grand Central Station, New York, NY 10163

Alcoholics have a prayer that helps them through difficult times. Study the prayer. It can be useful in everyone's life:

God grant me the serenity to accept the things I cannot change.
The courage to change the things I can.
The wisdom to know the difference.

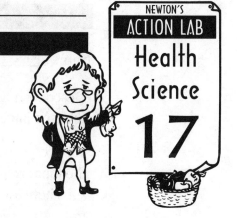

Investigating Tobacco

Dr. Newton Wants You to Know

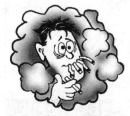

Every package of cigarettes carries this or a similar message.

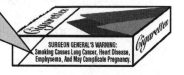

Surgeon General's Warning: Smoking Causes Lung Cancer, Heart Disease, Emphysema, And May Complicate Pregnancy.

Smoking can be smelly. Smoking can stain fingers and teeth. Smoking can affect breathing ability. Smoking can affect an athlete's endurance. Smoking can cause cancer and death.

So why do people still smoke? Dr. Newton wants you to take an opinion poll of smokers and non-smokers. Contact at least six people. Use the form below.

OCCUPATION	SMOKES-YES OR NO	THEIR OPINION ON SMOKING AND HEALTH

Tobacco Experiments

Tobacco Stains

1. Remove the filter and paper from two cigarettes.

2. Place the tobacco in a small baby food jar.

3. Add warm water so the jar is half full.

4. Wait 15 minutes.

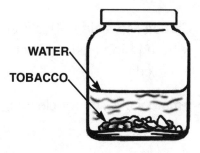

WATER

TOBACCO

Name _____

Describe how your tobacco juice looked and smelled. **Don't throw away your tobacco juice**.

Tobacco can stain your fingers and teeth. Prove this by placing a tooth substitute in the tobacco juice for three days. Use a piece of white chalk or white eggshell as your substitute tooth. Keep some extra chalk or eggshell outside the jar as a scientific control. After three days, compare the chalk or eggshell in the tobacco juice with the control group outside the jar.

Tobacco Chemicals

Burning tobacco releases dozens of chemicals. Some are harmless. Some are cancer-causing **carcinogen** chemicals.

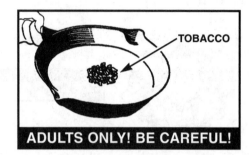

1. Remove the filter and paper from one cigarette.

2. Place the tobacco in a small metal pan.

Caution: Obtain adult help on the next step.

3. Heat the tobacco on a stove to release the chemicals.

4. Describe what you observe.

There are some strange, unpleasant chemicals coming from tobacco. Here are some of the chemicals you may have observed.

Tars: Blamed by some doctors as a cancer-causing carcinogen. Tar stains your teeth and fingers.

Aldehydes: Used in preservatives and disinfectants.

Glycerine: Used in medicines, cosmetics and explosives.

Here are some strange, unpleasant chemicals you could not have observed.

Nicotine: This is a **colorless** substance that can affect the circulatory, respiratory and digestive systems. Pure nicotine is a fatal **poison**.

Carbon Monoxide: This is also an invisible substance. It kills people by combining with red blood cells. Doctors blame the tiredness of chronic smokers on carbon monoxide.

Ammonia: Used for cleaning purposes.

58

Name _____

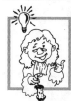

Building a Smoke Machine

1. Obtain a squeeze bottle or baster, a cigarette holder, some rubber tubing, cotton balls and a metal can.

2. Build the smoker shown on the right.

3. Place a **filter** cigarette in the holder.

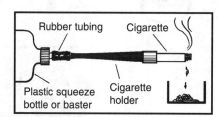

Rubber tubing   Cigarette

Plastic squeeze   Cigarette
bottle or baster   holder

Caution: You must have adult help to finish this experiment.

4. Squeeze the plastic bottle, and then have the adult light the cigarette. Work over the metal can. As you release the plastic bottle, smoke will flow into it.

5. **Slowly** squeeze and release the plastic bottle five times.

6. Remove the cigarette carefully and place it in the can.

7. Place a cotton ball over the end of the cigarette holder.

8. Squeeze the bottle five more times to force the smoke through the cotton ball.

9. Inspect the cotton ball and describe what you see.

10. Repeat the experiment using the same brand of cigarette but with the filter removed.

11. Compare the filter and non-filter cotton balls. Describe the differences, if any.

Dr. Newton Wants You to Advertise

You have just been given a job at a major advertising corporation. You have been assigned to prepare an antismoking radio commercial. Can you write a good antismoking ad? The facts below can help you.

TOBACCO FACTS

- One in four Americans smokes.
- Over three million people under the age of 18 smoke.
- Four in five smokers have tried to quit and failed.
- About 400,000 people die each year due to tobacco-related health problems.

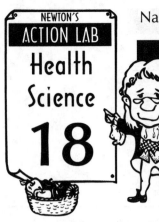

Name _____

Safety: Protect Your Precious Body

Dr. Newton Wants You to Think Safety

Dr. Newton wants you to live a long and healthy life. Among young people, accidents are a major cause of death and injury. You can avoid accidents in school, at home, at work or while driving by constantly thinking safety. Most accidents happen because of carelessness, fatigue and unsafe conditions in your environment.

ACCIDENT FACTS

- More teenagers die from accidents than disease.
- Young males have many more accidents than females.
- Over 10 million people are injured each year in accidents.
- Only heart disease, strokes and cancer cause more deaths than accidents.
- Home accidents cause over 30,000 deaths and four million injuries each year.
- Driving too fast is responsible for one-third of all auto deaths.

Dr. Newton Wants You to Think About Safety

1. Think about your last accident. How could it have been prevented?

2. What could you do to make your home safer?

3. What could be done to make school safer?

4. What could be done to make cars safer?

5. How could the sport of football be made safer?

Name _____

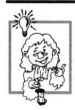

Dr. Newton's Safety Cartoon Contest

A good safety cartoon can teach safety better than a thousand words. Enjoy the safety cartoons below. Try to create a few safety cartoons of your own.

SAFETY CARTOONS

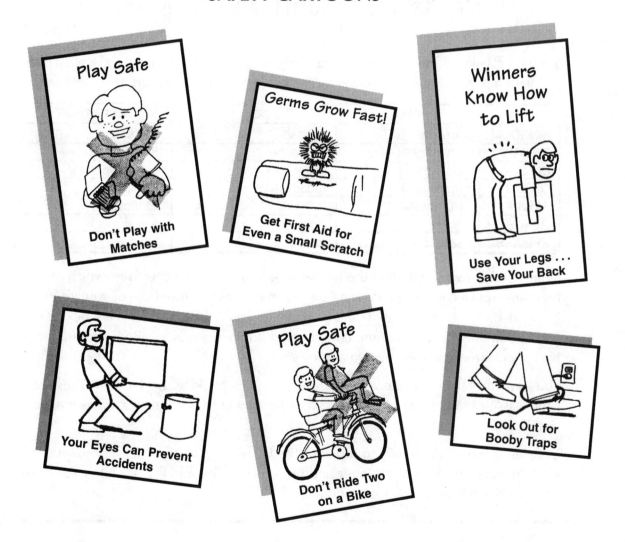

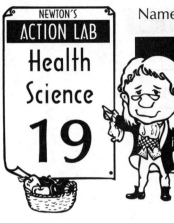

Name _____

Who Are You? Your Place in the Animal Kingdom

Dr. Newton Wants You to Know

Scientists classify and identify living things. They use Latin words so that the classified plant or animal has the same name all over the world. Here is a typical chart they might use.

	HUMAN	COW	WHITE PINE
KINGDOM	Animals	Animals	Plants
PHYLUM	Chordata	Chordata	Tacheophyta
CLASS	Mammalia	Mammalia	Gymnospermae
ORDER	Primates	Artiodactyla	Coniferales
FAMILY	Hominidae	Bovidae	Pinaceae
GENUS	*Homo*	*Bos*	*Pinus*
SPECIES	*sapiens*	*taurus*	*strobus*

Humans and cows are both in the animal kingdom. Both are **chordates** which means they have spinal chords. You and a cow are **mammals** because both of you are warm blooded, have hair, give birth to and feed milk to your young. Humans are next classified as **primates**. This leaves the cows behind but includes apes. Both you and apes have specialized arms and eyes in a bony socket.

You leave apes behind when you are classified as "Hominidae" or "Homo." These two Latin classifications mean "man-like." Your human species is called *sapiens* meaning "intelligent."

Congratulations. You are *Homo sapiens*. The white pine tree is *Pinus strobus*. Always start the genus with a capital letter and the species with a lowercase letter. Species names are generally in italics or underlined.

What's My Name?

You have a name that identifies you. Part of your name is the name of your entire family. Your friends all have names that identify them. Our world would be a confusing place without names.

Name _____

What is your dog's name? Dogs also have a Latin name. This Latin name is common for all kinds of dogs all over the world. Are you ready for this? Your dog's Latin name is *Canis familiaris.*

You will find the Latin names of some common plants and animals. Each name is followed by a clue. Can you identify them?

Latin Name	Clues	Common Names
1. *Equus caballus*	cowboy's best friend	_____
2. *Equus asinus*	looks like but isn't a horse	_____
3. *Schistocerca americana*	jumps around in the grass	_____
4. *Lumbricus terrestris*	crawls around inside the soil	_____
5. *Apis mellifera*	goes from flower to flower; an insect	_____
6. *Felis leo*	king of the beasts	_____
7. *Felis domestica*	has nine lives	_____
8. *Canis lupus*	Red Riding Hood had trouble with him	_____
9. *Homo sapiens*	a dog's best friend	_____
10. *Sequoia sempervirens*	giant California tree	_____
11. *Sibbaldus musculus*	largest mammal–found in the ocean	_____
12. *Melogris gallopavo*	very important during Thanksgiving	_____
13. *Syvilagus floridanus*	magicians pull him out of their hat	_____
14. *Castalia adorata*	common Easter flower	_____
15. *Mephitis mephitis*	animal with bad smell	_____

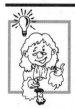

Dr. Newton Wants You to Classify Cars

Here is Dr. Newton's Latin classification for cars. Can you use it to classify your own cars or cars owned by your neighbors? Remember that you only need to work down from the class because all cars are in the kingdom **transportation** and the phylum **automobile**.

Kingdom	Phylum	Class	Order	Family	Genus	Species
transportation	automobile	domestic (American) or foreign	expensive medium inexpensive	year made (1900, 1995 or 1997)	make (Chevrolet, Buick, Honda, etc.)	model (convertible, station wagon, four-door, sedan, van, minivan or truck)

Dr. Newton drives a classy 1996 Buick convertible. Let's practice on his car.

Class: Domestic/**Order:** Expensive/**Family:** 1996/ **Genus:** Buick/**Species:** convertible

Its Latin name is *Buick convertible.* Now try some other cars.

Answer Key

Man's Marvelous Machine, page 8

1. air
2. move
3. grow
4. food
5. die
6. size
7. react
8. water
9. waste
10. repair
11. cells
12. protoplasm

How Long Can It Live? page 9

1. six weeks
2. two to six years
3. ten years
4. fifteen years
5. twenty years
6. seventy plus years
7. one hundred plus years
8. sixty years
9. ten years
10. thirty-five years
11. fifty years
12. forty-three years
13. fifty-eight years
14. seventy-nine years
15. seventy-two years
16. seventy-nine years
17. fifty-one years

Heredity Facts and Falsehoods, page 16

1. true
2. false
3. true
4. true
5. true
6. false
7. true
8. true
9. true

Dr. Newton Wants to Quiz You About Nutrition, page 28

All answers are true.